I0411327

Body Detox Brain Cleanse

Your Wellness PALS

Juicing and Smoothie Guide

Dr. Michael Wheat

Dedication

This book is dedicated to you, the reader. I honor your journey to Wellness and thank you for allowing me to be a small part of your success. Absorb, implement and have fun!

Common Sense Disclaimer

Medical Disclaimer:

I am not a medical doctor. I am a registered nurse and chiropractor with extensive, additional education in acupuncture, homeopathy and nutrition. The content expressed in my books, videos, and websites reflect personal experiences and ongoing research into functional, reversible conditions related to everyday health and nutrition.

The entire content of my books and websites isn't intended as a substitute for diagnosis or treatment. Always seek the advice of a qualified healer with any questions regarding a health condition, diagnosis, or a personalized treatment plan.

In case of medical emergency contact your doctor and/or call 911 immediately. Despite over a million reported medical errors that kill and injure hundreds of thousands of patients annually (according to the Journal of American Medical Association), calling 911 still beats calling the undertaker.

My Disclaimer:

Question everything including this content. Question the government, special interest groups and their agendas. Suit up and take responsibility for your own health. Educate yourself on what is truly best for you. Weigh your options and jump in. Live consciously. Love consciously. And eat consciously.

Acknowledgments

I would like to thank my family of origin and my family of choice. I thank my friends, acquaintances and especially my clients. Who I am today and what I offer here is a reflection of the lessons learned in previous iterations.

Cleanse Table of Contents

1 Introduction

Doing a cleanse gives your body-mind a break from its normal routine and the stressors you have placed upon it. Detoxification is a natural, automated process of your daily functioning. When you do a detoxification cleanse, you will take the overworked and stressed out body-mind back to its true and normal functioning. This is your optimal state and the way your body-mind is meant to be operating.

For some of you that are more toxic than others, this will be a little bumpy and feel like an accelerated pace as you may experience a healing episode. You will need to clean out the gutters to return to wellness and sometimes that job is messy. It will be my intention that you experience this part of your journey in the safest and easiest way possible.

The fact that you picked up this book tells that you are open-minded and willing to explore options. It tells me that you are looking for a positive, transformative healing. You are looking for wellness. It is through transformative healing that your innate power is released.

Know this. You are exactly where you are supposed to be; right here and right now. Being a culmination of your past choices, you represent today who you were. Some may cringe while others may celebrate. You are here by appointment. You are in the perfect right place.

You have a choice. Keep doing what you have always done and get what you have always gotten. Or start asking different questions and get different answers. The definition of insanity is doing the same thing over and over again expecting different results. If this is you, let's start asking different questions.

You may hear strange or foreign concepts. If you look deep enough they will resonate with you. If you experiment with the ideas in the book, I assure you wellness will follow. As with anything new, I encourage you to be open and follow the suggestions offered. Afterward, you can decide what serves you best.

Many times, the answers are right in front of us. We have only to allow and suspend any disbelief. Your intention for entering into a detoxification may be anything from feeling better to overcoming a significant challenge. The result for all of us however is functioning optimally and creating harmony in every aspect of our lives. Through proper nutrition the body hums like a well-oiled piece of machinery. And the brain works like a super computer. The soul receives downloads that are truly miraculous.

If you are one to avoid bumps along the road, you might want to start slow and progress as you see results. If you chose to jump in with both feet, you will progress much faster and can expect a little rockier road. There is no right or wrong way of doing anything including a cleanse. The right way is always your way!

I am grateful that you have chosen to spend a few hours with me and entertain the possibility of something greater in your life. I will endeavor to be gentle although some of you may feel like you have been hit by the proverbial cosmic 2x4.

2 Outcomes of a cleanse or detoxification

There are three outcomes of any cleanse or detoxification.

1.   You will get better.

2.   You will get better.

3.   And you will get better!

Having said this, let me explain further. Your body and your mind are meant to function optimally on living whole foods like Nature intended it. This means raw fruits, vegetables, nuts and seeds. These natural substances provide clean fuel and building blocks for your mind and body. Incorporating them into your daily routine is advisable. Fruits and vegetables are the bulk of what you will experience in any cleanse or detoxification program. However, this does not mean that you have to limit yourself to just these foods.

In the initial few cleanses, you will want to limit yourself to fruits, vegetables and potentially short list of other items. I would suggest that all your cleanses are fruits and vegetables. When you transition back to regular foods, please consider healthier choices and even trend toward an eighty percent raw diet with vegetable protein sources. I am getting ahead of myself here.

Let's consider the many benefits of a body-mind cleanse and a total detoxification program:

- Scrubbing and detoxifying your cells

- Repairing damaged cells

- Lowering blood pressure

- Lowering cholesterol

- Losing excess weight

- Losing stored toxins

  Slowing and reversing the aging process

- Regulating bowel activity

- Improving digestion

- Activating proper gene expression

- Increasing energy and rate of metabolism

- Igniting mental clarity

- Giving the body a much needed rest

- Eliminating abnormal changes

- Preventing more damage

- Improving body-mind efficiency

- Relieving tension

- Learning new eating habits

- Opening to spiritual downloads

- Creating greater intuition and body awareness

- Shifting into a new paradigm

- Busting through old patterns and limiting beliefs

- Engaging others more authentically

- Aligning with your higher purpose and vision

- Becoming who you are in your essence

3 Your Body-Mind Green Home

The Sun is an essential part of life. It is vital not only for plants but also for animals and humans. In fact, we need some amount of daily sunlight in the synthesis of vitamin D.

Plants absorb sunlight and convert it into energy through the chlorophyll molecule and a process called photosynthesis. Chlorophyll is what makes the plant green because of a central atom of magnesium. Chlorophyll is very similar to your own hemoglobin molecule in your blood. Hemoglobin carries oxygen in your red blood cells and delivers it into every cell in your body including your brain.

It is essential to utilize sunlight both directly and indirectly through plant consumption. As we eat plants, we are adding liquid sunshine to our body-mind system.

Consider your body-mind as an eco-friendly, green home. This home has many rooms for a variety of functions and various appliances that support a healthy environment and minimal impact on the surrounding ecosystem. It also represents minimal stress on your system.

This home is replete with solar panels, wind turbines, water purification and roof top gardening. It has a super bio-computer with a state of the art motherboard and intuitive technology that actually learns as it grows. And just wait until you hear about the stellar waste removal system!

Let's start at the top. The solar panels represent energy from the Sun being converted into useful energy for the house. It is the one thing that supports all other functions. This radiant heat and energy supplies directly to the body and also is utilized for your rooftop gardens.

Wind turbines can be thought of as fresh air needed to sustain life. Again, wind adds another essential component in your body-mind household. Your water filtration system allows for only the freshest water to enter the body and is needed only when superior water cannot be sourced. Water is utilized to run all internal operations of your household as well as the garden up top. Water is vital for life.

Ah, the garden. This rooftop garden is the beginning point for all nutritional sustenance. There is some soil based and some hydroponic gardening in constant flux. It is an organic garden full of lush vegetation, both fruits and vegetables. There are vegetables and fruits representing all colors of the rainbow. This is a sanctuary of variety, goodness and wholesomeness. It is a great place to meditate and set intentions for the day. It fuels your day on many levels.

The produce from the garden will consist of everything you need to run your household. Consider the leafy, green vegetables chalk full of proteins to be the tools needed to build and repair your home. Fruits could represent the furniture and artwork that makes your home nice and cozy. All this vegetation is processed into liquid sunshine that is used as a biofuel for the body-mind home.

Each room in the home represents different functional areas. You have a kitchen to process food and a den where all the business of the household gets done. The den is a place for the business of your life. There must be a recreation room for play and of course a bedroom for amazing sleep. There is a room solely dedicated to processing and handling waste from your home.

All these rooms and the operations of all activities are governed by the master control room, your bio-computer or brain. The brain is nothing more than a super user computer. It is able to process information and run algorithms at lightening speeds. It is able to leverage past events to 'think' and provide new solutions in an ever-changing world. It is part of the body.

The mind is something quite different. The brain is like a processor while the mind is the abstract, intellectual aspect and encompasses higher level soul functions. More on this in another book.

The entire body-mind household utilizes the sun, wind and water directly and indirectly through the garden. Garden produce converted into liquid sunshine biofuel delivers energy directly to the household.

All this is to say that your body-mind needs direct sunlight, fresh air, pristine water and wholesome, unaltered food for clean living and minimal impact. The more you deviate from this the more out of balance you become, within your body-mind and within the great plan of Nature.

These four elements of natural living are consistent in every culture to some degree. As you tamper with Nature's design by introducing less than optimal nutrition, imbalances will occur. The body-mind system is a wonderful self-correcting mechanism. It will adjust and adjust until it becomes overwhelmed and then it 'breaks down'. This is when symptoms arrive. The imbalance has been occurring for some time as the body attempted to adjust.

The body must purge and reboot. This is what illness and detoxification looks like. They actually are one in the same process albeit aspects of the same continuum. Like detoxification, an illness is an attempt to rid the body of toxins. What is perceived as illness are various forms of roadblocks set up to slow you down enough for the body to initiate a detoxification program.

Right nutrition and proper detoxification are the keys to a successfully run body-mind green household that functions optimally and adapts quickly to changing conditions.

4 Toxicity

Right nutrition and effective detoxification are the two essential ingredients to a healthy, long life. The body is in a constant, dynamic state. This is called homeostasis and keeps the body in balance with opposing forces, like bringing in nutrients to the cells for proper functioning and eliminating waste products. There are many other examples within the millions of body-mind processes that could be listed here.

Think of this like the ebb and flow of waves in the ocean. It is important to have good nutrition coming in and proper waste removal going out. If there is less than optimal nutrition in the body it will not function properly. It is equally true that substandard waste removal will result in an accumulation of toxins and poorer health.

Poor nutrition and poor elimination result in toxicity. Toxicity on some level is a part of or solely responsible for each and every illness or health condition you will ever experience. When you tackle these two elements concurrently, your health will soar to the heights of wellness quickly.

It should be common sense at this point that fast food is not proper nutrition. There are of course many other more subtle food sources that are not what could be considered proper nutrition. For example, processed food stuffs and many sweets are poisons to your body-mind and should be marginalized if not completely eliminated from your diet. I know. I hate the word 'should' as well. I hate toxicity even more!

So hang in there. Once you are clean and clear, you will start to feel the same way and may even become a detox nut. Let's just agree to cleanse for now. We can deconstruct or revamp your diet later. I told you I would be gentle…

There are a couple of results that occur from poor nutrition and improper waste removal. When you become toxic, your body is unable to keep up with the appropriate level of waste removal. You get backed up and bogged down. You start to develop symptoms and show signs of illness, dis-ease and low level functioning. Eventually, your brain functions at a lower level and you become unable to process information, make congruent decisions or focus on higher level desires. You are in a rut and there is no light at the end of that tunnel.

You soon begin to spiral downward as inappropriate food and drink choices become the norm. You generally crave these dreadful choices more and more. These cravings will continue to toxify your body-mind. You tend to over eat as a way to bring in what little nutrition is available in cooked or processed food stuffs. Overeating and obesity are definite signs of toxicity. For those of you on the thinner side, make no mistake as you may be even more toxic.

When you over eat carbohydrates, you experience intoxication like drinking alcohol. This actually lulls you into a sense of comfort however this is a very dangerous scenario. As you over eat meats and proteins, these sit in your gut for extended periods of time and putrefy. Putrefaction is decomposition of organic matter. It is not a bad thing generally in nature however in your gut this process releases toxins. These toxins are absorbed through your intestinal wall. The longer the meat sits there the more toxins are released into your body-mind.

This is the proverbial hamster in the wheel and you don't even know you are there. You will make poorer and poorer choices and end up with chronic dis-eases, physically and mentally. Your emotions are whack at this point! This is a sad state indeed and you are not alone. Many people suffer under the same toxic yoke.

Stop the insanity. This is getting quite depressing. Let's shift gears and talk about what happens on the lighter side of nutrition. As you make optimal food and drink choices, you actually tonify your body-mind. This means health and healing. This means a trend toward wellness and wholeness. Now we are talking!

As you detox and cleanse you return to health and your energy on all levels soars. When the body has proper nutrition it responds rapidly and you will be amazed as to how well…and different you feel. This is the whole purpose of detoxification. Your elimination organs have been working overtime just their spinning wheels. You were exhausting vital energy resources and were becoming exhausted. Now you have breathing space to dump the toxic overload and return to vibrancy.

Initially, the cleanse will relieve the body-mind of this toxic stress because you are bringing in proper nutrition, actually super-sized nutrition. Although you are taking right action, the road may be a bit bumpy. Depending on your level of toxicity, you may experience symptoms of detoxification. Do not confuse illness with your toxic overload symptoms. A subsequent chapter will discuss this topic in more depth.

When you return to a higher level of functioning and stay there, you will be tonifying your body-mind. This is a phenomenal state where you get to experience health and wellness. You will feel better, think clearer and be much happier. You will be able to access inspiration and creativity more readily.

5 What is a cleanse or detox program?

When you choose to cleanse your body-
mind system, you are fasting from your
normal dietary intake and detoxifying. This
means that you are eliminating toxins that
have built up over time and need removal.
As previously stated, this is a normal
process under normal conditions. When you
become toxic and exhibit symptoms, you
have already placed way too much stress on
your waste removal system. It is in hyper
drive and not only needs to catch up but also
needs to take a break. Detoxing gives your
body-mind that break.

A true fast is having nothing to eat for a
period of time. This means water only. You
may have noticed that animals often do not
eat when sick. This is a natural process to
allow the immune system to focus on
healing and not on breaking down toxic
processed foods. Water fasting alleviates
your entire system of the burden you have
placed upon it with substandard nutritional
choices. A true fast can be and is generally
stressful for the uninitiated simply because it
is such a drastic contrast to the usual, dietary

intake. Here is an opportunity to be gentle with yourself and ease into your first detox. If this is old hat for you then choose to deepen into a more substantive detox…with grace and ease.

If you have not done a water fast before, I would suggest that you ease into it with a juice cleanse. Juicing allows you to be partially or totally satiated and will ultimately accomplish the same result. It is safer and slower to juice your way to better health. And juice detoxification is the focus of this book.

Juicing for a cleanse is ease and fun. You will have an opportunity to experiment with various fruits and vegetables and see what you really like. You will also play around with how long you want to stay in the detox mode. There will be general guidelines proposed here, however you are the ultimate authority on what works best for you.

In general, a cleanse increases the amount of fruits, vegetables and water that you might normally have in your diet. There are some of you that eat no fruits or vegetable so consider yourself on notice. You will be increasing your fruit and vegetable intake by 100% or more. There may be a few additional items that are part of the detox solution for you. These recommendations will be outlined in subsequent chapters.

You may choose to juice all your fruits and vegetables removing the pulp or fiber. This is a superb way to approach a cleanse as you get mega doses of rich nutrients into your body-mind system quickly with ease of assimilation. Utilizing a smoothie approach retains the fiber and for some is preferable. Smoothies have needed soluble and insoluble fiber that efficiently cleans and scrubs the colon. Where you may juice 20 carrots in a day, you may not eat that amount of carrots in a smoothie. So smoothies are a great way to self- regulate.

Regardless, know that on the juice or smoothie detox program with the right nutrition you will not need to worry about overconsumption. Most people have been overeating with the wrong nutrients. So 'overeating' with the right nutrients at least while on the cleanse is a welcome change as it loads your deficient nutrient account with needed vitamins, minerals, co-factors and living water. When you add right nutrition your body-mind responds accordingly and will take exactly what it needs discarding the rest and sending 'shut off' instructions to the brain.

If you are doing an extended cleanse and are hungry in the first couple of days, the hunger is a reflection of the body memory with eating at certain times of the day. Simply add more juices and it should curb your appetite. Those extending longer than three days will experience the disappearance of hunger altogether for days, weeks or months during the cleanse. Yes, I said months. You can live for months without food. Again, this is not the focus of this book. Extended fasts are best reserved for the experienced or supervised.

When true hunger returns as well as a few other indicators, it is time to end the cleanse. You may notice a coating on your tongue and when it clears again this is a sign that the detox is ending. Your body-mind will only release toxins at a certain rate. When it is done for the moment, hunger will return and you will be ready to transition off the detox juices. If you extend the detox or fast beyond the return of true hunger, you will be entering starvation and this of course is unhealthy.

The more you ease into and out of the core portion of the cleanse, the more comfort you will experience. The more toxic you are and the quicker you accelerate the detox, the more uncomfortable you will be. This discomfort is temporary and not severe. Believe me, you are far more uncomfortable now and have simply adapted to it. So you assume that you are OK. However, you are likely far from OK at the cellular level. If you have been slamming fast food three times a day and jump cold turkey into a water fast, you will likely trigger what is known as a healing event or a healing episode. Some call the extreme ones healing crises. Let's avoid a crisis if at all possible. Ease in and ease out. Got it?

What may be unavoidable is the fact that you could experience detox symptoms. These mimic cold and flu-like symptoms.

Why? Because every illness whether acute or chronic, uses the same organs of elimination that you will be using as you detox. In fact, every acute or chronic dis-ease is a detox. It is an attempt by the body to remove the toxicity, right the wrongs and take the stressors away.

The nature of dis-ease is the scope of another book. Suffice it to say for now that you have a toxic build up and are unable to remove it efficiently which will lead to more complications in the future. When is *now* a good time to trend back to wellness? Juice detoxing is a sure fire way to jumpstart your recovery and sets you on that road to wellness. Juice, eliminate toxins and be well! NOW!

6 Methods of Elimination and Detox

When you enter into a detox program, your body-mind goes into dump mode as it purifies itself and eliminates its toxic build up. There may be few symptoms or there may be several. Your body will use its organs of elimination to remove toxins. You may also experience mental and emotional symptomology as the toxins recirculate through your bloodstream and brain on their way out of the kidneys.

The five major organs of elimination are the gastrointestinal tract, the kidneys, the lungs, the liver and the skin. As you begin your detox, these organs will begin to accelerate their respective toxin releases. Remember that the more toxic you are the more you may experience detox symptoms. If they become uncomfortable, simply back off your program a bit. Slow down or shorten your program. If you need to back off, that should be a red flag for you that you are quite toxic and really need a cleanse. You may want to do more frequent and shorter cleanses until you can manage a detox with little or no symptomology. We will discuss a maintenance schedule later.

As a precautionary note, some of your old suppressed symptoms may reappear or escalate. Remember the body uses the same routes in illness and in detoxification. If you find yourself becoming symptomatic, check in with yourself. It is important to continue the detox and not medicate yourself. You are dumping toxic chemicals including medications and do not want to reintroducing them. Again, slow down by having a very light meal like steamed vegetables or an apple until the discomfort subsides. It is preferable to simply ride out the storm. You will be doing short cleanses in the beginning and your body-mind will soon adapt to detox sessions.

You may experience general symptoms to some degree. Mild headaches are quite common. The dull, achy types are the norm. The pain relates to toxins being dumped into the bloodstream and circulated throughout the body and brain before elimination. Weakness or lethargy is common as well. Your body is focused on cleaning and diverts energy internally. Less energy is available for strenuous activity and strength. Achy muscles and flu-like symptoms may appear as toxins work their way out of your musculature. Get a massage. Body temperature tends to decreased on a cleanse. So bundle up!

The lungs will release toxic gases trapped in the blood during normal respiration. In detox mode, the lungs off gas chemicals and natural substances at different rates to balance your body as the other elimination organs remove the trash. You may sense a change in respiratory rates or getting 'winded' easily. Take it slow and dial back on activity during a detox. You are shifting gears from external activity to internal cleansing activity. Your body needs to focus and not be overstimulated.

The liver is a major internal player. You will not notice many symptoms here either although this is where the lion's share of toxins reside and need to purge through the bile duct into the gastrointestinal tract for expulsion. The liver converts or plays a role in the conversion of every process in your body. If it identifies toxins often times it will sequester them. Your liver is like the oil filter on your car. The difference is that your liver never gets changed. So you have to clean it internally with cleanses. You may experience discomfort over your liver area (right side at and below your ribcage) and deep within the right side of your abdomen. Supplementation, massage and manual manipulation of the liver will help reduce this discomfort. As the detox progresses, any discomfort will subside.

Your gastrointestinal tract runs from your mouth through your stomach and into your small intestines and colon to exit via the rectum and anus. The tract is one long tube truly outside your body although it appears to be internal. As food and drink move along its length nutrients and living water are absorbed. The GI tract makes every attempt to absorb only nutritious substances and even has mechanisms to eliminate toxins quickly. The challenge is when only garbage is coming in, the tract absorbs everything of value it can. The downside is that it picks up toxins as well. If you eat all natural, raw and organic food stuffs, your body-mind would not get toxic.

As you detox, all the gunk, grit, grime and slime begin to break free and are expelled. This means you will likely experience freedom from constipation and even diarrhea. This is your body dumping toxins at an accelerated rate. No need to worry, just hydrate. You may have bloating and gas as well as a bit of nausea. The nausea may be two fold; from the toxic release and from the change in diet because of lower blood sugar. Please note that juices provide more than adequate nutrition just less calories than most are used to eating. If nauseated, add more juices as you can tolerate them. Give your gut a free ride with enemas and colonics. Be wise with your usage of colonics or enemas and hydrate.

One of the hallmark signs of detoxification is a coated tongue. Your tongue will get coated and possibly discolored. The more gunk on the tongue, the more toxic you are. The tongue is an indicator of what is happening all along your GI tract. This is real work being done here. As you might imagine, you will have foul breath as well. Use something natural if you are offensive. Do not use a chemical mouth wash. Chew on some mint leaves and remember when the tongue clears so does the gut. For the moment...

Skin is the largest toxic organ. Every single little pore is a possible toxic removal site. So this means your skin may get pimples, rashes or other lesions. This is a great sign that you are eliminating toxins. Once this clears you will see beautifully renewed and vibrantly healthy skin unlike you have even seen before. Don't put anything on your skin that you would not eat. Ouch! Anyone out there using cosmetics please take heed. I have a shoulder you can cry on. And while you are at it, grab a loofah or a pair of those cool skin massage gloves and starting scrubbing. Working the dead skin off and opening the pores is great for your skin and your detox program.

Your kidneys will handle the brunt of toxic liquids they filter from your bloodstream. You want to make sure your kidneys are in good working order. The more you pee the more you flush those toxins out and the less discomfort you will experience. There are a host of supportive herbs for the kidneys. Drinking distilled water will greatly assist with the removal of liquid waste. It will pull toxins out of your bloodstream at an alarming rate.

With all this body talk, I would be remiss if I left out your psychological welfare. Restricting one's diet and doing a cleanse takes dedication and will power. It can be a bit overwhelming at the onset and you may feel all alone. This time can also bring up past emotions that need to be purged as well. Let them go and know that you are doing something positive for yourself. The return on your invest will be well worth it. Hang in there and seek supportive friends, family or organizations.

Along with the mental game, you may actually have cause for some of the other disturbances. Since the toxins will be flowing, you may experience irritability or anxiousness. Some of these toxins are excitatory and can get you revved up in a negative way. Ride it out while you flush it

out. Remember the distilled water. You may
have difficulty sleeping or odd cravings.
Pain is technically a psychological beast and
can be overridden with some practice. Try
meditation, yoga or nature walks. The
discomfort will subside.

Next up is a healing episode.

7 The Healing Episode

Anytime there is a shift in routine there will also be a shift in outcomes. When you choose to cleanse, you will have toxins jumping ship. This means that the toxins have to disengage from whence they have been hiding or stuck and circulate out of your body-mind system. They will all circulate through the blood or bowel as they find their respective exit routes.

Anything lodged in the bowel will move out through the bowel sometimes at an accelerated rate with the assistance of juices and smoothies. The smoothies will carry broom-sweeping soluble and insoluble fibers that attract and expel toxic build up in the gut. Allow me to be graphic for a moment. Some individuals have certain food items that they have not been consumed for weeks, months or even years released through the bowel. Now I would call that quite toxic. Remember that carb overload produces fermentation and protein overload putrefies in the gut. Can you say 'yuck'?

The blood system is a remarkable system in the body. The elimination organs are anxiously awaiting the circulatory system to unload its dangerous, hazardous cargo. The lungs release toxic vapors from the blood while the kidneys filter all the water soluble vermin. The skin expels solids and liquids from third spacing and plugged pores. The liver does the conversions and then dumps solid waste into the gut and out through the bowel. The blood circulates the rest of the liver toxins.

The circulation of toxic blood can cause symptoms. As well, anything moving from a stuck location through one of the elimination organs can produce symptomology. In the previous chapter, we looked at some of those rascals and a few comfort measures. Here we will address the big event…

There are times within a detox cycle that you may experience an aggravation of old symptoms or a spike in discomfort. Again, that may be signs like the flu, headaches, pains or any number of others unique to you. It is important to carefully assess these signs and symptoms before making any rash decisions. Do not be quick to end your cleanse.

When experiencing a healing episode or event, check in frequently throughout the exacerbation and mentally remind yourself why you started this in the first place. I want to remind you the more discomfort the more toxicity in your body-mind. Don't let a little discomfort dissuade you from your mission!

When the event becomes quite uncomfortable you may be experiencing a healing crisis. It sounds really bad, doesn't it? Well it is not. It is simply darned uncomfortable. Pull on you big girl panties or big boy pants. This is when you need to be more motivated and more present than at any other time. Trust the process and trust your body. It knows what it is doing.

We talked about two very important milestones when ending a detox cycle. Clearing of the tongue and the return of true hunger are those milestones. So let's dig a little deeper. You are sucking down your green smoothies. You are experiencing headaches and they are getting quite painful.

You have a little annoying diarrhea and a few unsightly pimples. Your tongue is coated and your breath stinks. No one will kiss you. Do you continue the cleanse or throw in the towel?

Of course you continue. And I promise that after the detox, everyone will want to kiss you especially as you share your success story. Remember, true hunger is the body telling you it is time to eat. True hunger is not following the clock or your companions to happy hour. When your tongue clears, you have the green light to get social (wink).

OK, so what do you do when experiencing a healing event? Firstly, as previously mentioned get present and assess the situation. Make a judgment call as to whether this is something you can manage or need assistance to process. If you chose to move forward, back off a little from your current routine and be nice to yourself. Don't get too aggressive at this point. If you choose to take a break from the detox, you need to be very cautious. Absolutely, do not run to the nearest buffet. Not only will this reverse every good thing you have accomplished but also may be dangerous.

The easiest way to break the detox and to avoid problems is to reintroduce solid foods slowly over a couple of days. I suggest that if you are juicing that you move to smoothies for a day or two advancing to high water content fruits like citrus, grapes, tomatoes or cucumbers. From there you can move into light salads and beyond. Eating only one fruit or vegetable at a time can be helpful as well. There is no need to worry about quantity at this point. After a couple of days, you may start to add additional healthy choices. Hopefully, you have had time to consider not returning to some of your old toxic favorites.

If you are doing smoothies, pick up with the whole fruits and advance to veggies. After the first few days of using smoothies, it is highly unlikely that you well have any untoward symptoms. In fact, weight loss and toxin release should keep you trekking down the detox road. How long? That is entirely up to you and the topic of a subsequent chapter.

As a general rule, healing events are mild and manageable. When they get wily, ease off the accelerator a bit and regroup. If you feel you need to continue and have concerns, reach out for assistance preferably to someone with experience in detoxification. Once you have been through the detox gauntlet, you will know your own threshold and will push the envelope a bit.

Healing events are a good sign that you are dumping that toxic load. Let it go and be grateful!

8 Detoxification and Cleanse Protocols

This is the 'nuts and bolts' chapter. Here you will learn how to implement a cleanse. We will be discussing equipment needed, general supplies and specific protocols. You will also make decisions on the length, intensity level, day of the week to begin and type of detox with which you will want to start.

Let's talk about equipment. You will need a cutting board and a sharp knife. The larger the knife the less wear and tear on your hands especially if you are not used to preparing meals and/or chopping large volumes of fruits and vegetables. You will want to invest in a blender and a juicer. Both can be found at your local box store for very little cash outlay. You do not need a $500 blender although it will certainly make the smoothies smoother and is worth the investment someday. Likewise, having a $400 juicer will extract more vital juices and nutrients however unnecessary in the beginning. Follow the use and cleaning instructions for both devices.

If you choose to use a cheap blender and your smoothies are chunkier than desired, you can strain through a colander or cheese cloth to elimination the chunks and some of the fiber. When you decide on juicing versus smoothies or a combination then you will decide on chunky versus smooth. That does not mean peanuts butter, folks!

As for supplies, this is your decision. The goal is to get as many detoxifying elements into your cleanse as possible. Fruits and vegetable fit this bill nicely. Feel free to use standard items that you may consume on a regular basis. This will give you some comfort since you are familiar with the tastes of them. However, the sky is the limit so experiment. Any fruits and vegetables will work. You will want to use both fruits and vegetables especially leafy green vegetables like lettuces, kales, chards and spinach.

You will have a couple of options when it comes to start dates and lengths of cleanses. I would suggest a short three day detox and starting on a Friday (or your weekend). It likely will be your last day of work week and you could muddle through the day with juice only. You might get a little hungry and headachy later in the day. Remember the more toxic the more detox symptoms you may experience. The bulk of your detox will happen over your weekend and with less activity should be less stressful. You and your body can focus on the detox and not having to concentrate on work.

I would suggest you start with smoothies if it is your first time and you feel as though you are quite toxic. Otherwise, jump into a juicing protocol. It is only three days. You will manage just fine. And you will be checking in with yourself throughout the weekend to see if you need to adjust anything in your protocol. Do a simply check in. Am I OK? Do I need anything right now? Then appreciate the cleanse work you have done thus far, even if it is only a couple of hours.

The basic smoothie recipe is very simple and easy. In a blender, add two pieces of fruit or cups of chopped fruit or berries along with two large handfuls of leafy green vegetables. Fill up the blender with greens.

Add a little distilled water and blend until smooth. Then add additional distilled water up to one quart or liter and spin. This little trick will minimize chunks. Also using softer fruits and vegetables will minimize chunks as well. Clean-up is a breeze. Just rinse and repeat with your blender carafe.

The basic juice recipe is pretty much the same with about a 50/50 ratio of fruits and vegetables. You will need more volume though because you are juicing and this removes all the fiber. This juice will be concentrated and can be enjoyed as is or diluted. You have been running on empty nutritionally so during the cleanse you may consume as much juice as you want without concern. Some programs require up to 15-20 glasses of juice per day. The juicer clean-up is a little more labor intensive but well worth it.

Whether you choose the basic smoothie or basic juice protocol, both will have profound effects for you. I would suggest sticking with one so you can evaluate the results. Next time you can switch it up. You will want to review the basic recipes in the next chapters, invent your own or refer to our companion recipe guide. The point is to rest your gut, supply ample nutrients and remove as many toxins as possible throughout the duration of your cleanse.

Let's talk a bit more about length of a cleanse. There are some proponents of a weekly day fast. Some religious groups might choose a Sunday and others may use a Monday after a weekend of indulgence. When you abstain from food and drink for a day it gives your body time to rest. This process will take longer to detox but is gentler than other programs. It is also a good maintenance practice. Some like a three day detox every month to three months. Three days of cleansing will really get the toxins moving out.

Others will do a 10-14 day fast once per year or bi-annually during the spring and fall. This is a wonderful experience as your body shifts from a winter diet to a summer diet in the spring and of course the opposite in the fall. When you are really in tune with your body-mind consider this as a superior option. Then there are the wild ones that just go for it. You can live on water only for months and certainly indefinitely on juices or smoothies. Again, if you are going to do an extended detox it should not be your first and it should be supervised. See our long fast book on the longer protocols.

9 Detox Protocols

Day of the Week Cleanse

Pick a day each week that is conducive and relatively stress free.

Refrain from regular diet and drink only distilled water OR prepare fresh juices/smoothies for the day.

Repeat weekly.

Observe and record what happens on that day and over time.

The Three Day Detox

Pick a day that is most appropriate to start and minimize activity during detox.

Go shopping the day before so you have the freshest, organic produce available.

Get up a little earlier that day to prepare your first juice or smoothie.

Rinse fruits and vegetable so they are free of any visible dirt. It is OK for you to consume a few microbes. They are good for you.

Chop fruits and vegetable to fit into your machine. Many can be used whole.

It is best to consume immediately after processing your fresh juice or smoothie. However, it may not be practical. If you need to blend juice for the day, it is acceptable. If you can juice or blend before you need each drink, all the better.

During the three days, observe and record what happens on those days.

Adjust accordingly. If you are juicing and need to slow down, prepare a smoothie or eat an apple. Then return to juice later in the day.

<u>The Seven to Ten Day Detox</u>

Extend the Three Day Detox

The difference here is a much longer cleanse and a much deepen detoxification.

This is a great length of time to incorporate enemas or colonics.

Watch yourself closely and record your results.

10 Fresh Juice Recipes

<u>Basic Citrus Juice</u>

Any citrus or combination of citrus

Peel citrus and run through juicer.

<u>Basic Detox Juice</u>

Equal portions of leafy greens and fruits

Run through juicer.

<u>Basic Chelation Juice</u>

Basic Detox recipe with additional parsley and/or cilantro

Run through juicer.

<u>Basic Fruit Juice</u>

Any fruits except bananas (they don't juice well at all. Add them to your smoothie recipes)

Run through juicer.

Basic Root Juice

Carrots will be your base

Add beets as desired

Add other roots vegetable as desired

Run through juicer.

Basic Vegetable Juice

Tomato and/or carrot as a base

Add celery, onion, bell pepper, leafy greens, cucumber or any other vegetable as desired

Run through juicer.

Basic Sprout Juice

Add 1 -2 boxes or 4-8 ounces of sprouts to any juice recipe

Run through juicer.

Basic Green Juice

Leafy greens (chards, lettuces, kales, cabbages, herbs, etc)

Apple as desired to cut bitterness

Run through juicer.

Basic Melon Juice

(melon juices should be enjoyed alone)

Any melon or combination or melons

Slice, deseed and cube for juicing. Run through juicer.

Basic Apple Juice

Apples

Add small amount of ginger root, lime, lemon or any other complement for variety

Run through juicer.

11 Fresh Smoothie Recipes

Basic Detox Smoothie

2 fruits or equivalent (apple, banana, berries, citrus, etc)

2 large handfuls of leafy greens or sprouts

Combine all ingredients in blender with minimal distilled water or other appropriate liquid. Blend until smooth and thick. Add water or other liquid to one quart/liter and blend again. Drink in one setting or enjoy throughout the morning before other foods are consumed.

Basic Chelation Detox Smoothie

2 fruits or equivalent (apple, banana, berries, citrus, etc)

1 large handful of leafy greens or sprouts

1 bunch cilantro or parsley

Garlic cloves to taste (optional)

Combine all ingredients in blender with minimal distilled water or other appropriate liquid. Blend until smooth and thick. Add water or other liquid to one quart/liter and blend again. Drink in one setting or enjoy throughout the morning before other foods are consumed.

Basic Berry Smoothie

6-8 oz fresh or flash frozen berries

1-2 apples

Combine all ingredients and blend until smooth.

Basic Root Smoothie

2 carrots

1 beet

1 potato, sweet potato or yam

1-2 stalks of celery

1 bunch parsley

Garlic cloves to taste

Distilled water to thin as desired

Combine all ingredients and blend until smooth.

Basic Green Protein Smoothie

2 handfuls of spinach, kale or other dark leafy green

2 stalks of celery

1-2 cucumbers

1-2 teaspoons spirulina or other algae (optional)

1-2 apples for sweetness (optional)

Combine all ingredients and blend until smooth.

Basic Vegetable Smoothie

1-2 carrots

1-2 green onions

1 handful of leafy greens

2-4 tomatoes

1-2 cucumbers

1 bell pepper

1-2 stalks of celery

1 pinch of hot pepper powder (optional)

Combine all ingredients and blend until smooth.

Basic Sprout Smoothie

1-2 boxes of sprouts

1-2 pieces of fruit or berries

Combine all ingredients and blend until smooth. Add distilled water to desired thickness.

Basic Nut Mylk Smoothie

2-4 oz of nuts or seeds

1 quart/liter of distilled water, coconut water or other appropriate liquid

Add nuts or seeds to blender with small amount of liquid. Blend until smooth then add remainder or liquid. This mylk can be substituted for distilled water in any recipe.

Basic Citrus Recipe

2-4 citrus fruits (oranges, grapefruits, tangerines, combination, etc)

1 bunch red clover sprouts or other mild sprouts (optional but you better try it)

Peel citrus. Combine all ingredients and blend until smooth.

Basic Melon Recipe

(melons should be consumed alone)

½-1 melon depending on size (watermelon, cantaloupe, honeydew, etc)

Cut melon, remove seeds and cube flesh. Combine all ingredients and blend until smooth.

Basic Fat Supplements

Good Fats: Add young coconut water and pulp to any recipe

Good Fats: Add 1-2 teaspoons of extra virgin olive oil, hemp oil or any appropriate good fat to any recipe

Good Fats: Add ½ to 1 avocado to any recipe

Good Fats: Add 1-2 oz of nuts or seeds as desired to any recipe

Resources

www.purelifegreens.com

www.mindimpress.com

www.yourwellnesspals.com

Hamlyn, *Juices and Smoothies*

Meyerowitz, Steve, *Juice Fasting and Detoxification*

Carrington, Hereward, *Fasting for Health and Long Life*